Sabrine Louhaichi
Besma Hamdi

Bronchiolitis obliterans in children

Sabrine Louhaichi
Besma Hamdi

Bronchiolitis obliterans in children

Clinical and functional impact of therapeutic management in a pediatric pulmonary unit

ScienciaScripts

Imprint

Cover image: www.ingimage.com

This book is a translation from the original published under ISBN 978-620-6-71836-9.

Publisher:
Sciencia Scripts
is a trademark of
Dodo Books Indian Ocean Ltd. and OmniScriptum S.R.L publishing group

120 High Road, East Finchley, London, N2 9ED, United Kingdom
Str. Armeneasca 28/1, office 1, Chisinau MD-2012, Republic of Moldova, Europe
Printed at: see last page
ISBN: 978-620-8-32614-2

To my teacher and jury president Professor Sleheddine Chouchène

You have done us the honour of agreeing to chair this jury and evaluate this work. Please accept the expression of our profound gratitude for your availability and kindness.

To my teacher and jury member Professor Saoussen Cheikh Mhamed

We would like to thank you very much for your availability and extreme kindness. We thank you for the honor you have bestowed on us by agreeing to sit on the jury.

To my teacher and jury member Professor Najeh Ben Fadhel

We are deeply honored by your presence on the jury for our dissertation. Please accept our deepest respect.

To my teacher and thesis supervisor Professor Besma Hamdi

I had the privilege of having you as my study director. Your scientific rigor and kindness were an invaluable contribution to this work. May this work be an expression of my profound gratitude.

Signing sessions

To my teacher, Professor Agnès Hamzaoui, you inspired the subject of this work. Your advice, guidance and meticulousness have made an invaluable contribution to my development. Your scientific rigor, your passion for this noble profession and your immense dedication have left a lasting impression on me. I would like to express my deep gratitude and I hope to live up to the trust you have placed in me.

To my teacher Dr Jamel Ammar, it's been a real honor and an enriching experience to learn from you. Your advice and encouragement have guided me through this beautiful specialty. I dedicate this work to you as a token of my deep gratitude.

To all the medical and paramedical staff of Pneumology Department B at Abderrahmen Mami Hospital in PAriana It's a real pleasure to work with your dedicated team every day, and I'd like to express my gratitude and thanks.

Table of contents

INTRODUCTION

Bronchiolitis obliterans (BO) in children is a chronic inflammatory disease of the airways. The disease most often occurs following severe pulmonary infection or bone marrow transplantation as part of graft-versus-host disease (GVHD). Much more rarely, it may be due to connective tissue disease (1).

Positive diagnosis combines several clinical, functional and radiological elements (2). However, the performance of respiratory function tests depends on the child's age and cooperation.

The prognosis of BO depends on etiology, early positive diagnosis and therapeutic management (3). The course of the disease can be marked by a number of complications, including chronic respiratory failure and pulmonary hypertension.

Admittedly, this is a rare respiratory pathology compared with other chronic childhood lung diseases such as asthma. However, its management poses a real public health challenge, given the high morbidity and mortality associated with it and the absence of a therapeutic consensus (4).

Therapeutic protocols for small series of children with BO have been reported in the literature, with controversial results. The most commonly used molecules were macrolides, anti-leukotrienes, inhaled bronchodilators and inhaled or systemic corticosteroids (5).

In developing countries, there is a delay in diagnosing this pathology, given the difficulties of monitoring children's respiratory function following severe respiratory infections or bone marrow transplants.

Moreover, even after a positive diagnosis, the management of BO in our context may not be optimal. Indeed, the difficulty of access to care facilities for these patients, on the one hand, and the non-availability of certain drugs in hospitals, on the other, hamper the prognosis of the disease in these children (6).

To this end, we set out to study the clinical and paraclinical profile of children followed in our department for obliterative bronchiolitis, and to assess the impact of our management on the clinical and functional prognosis of the disease.

METHODS

I. Type of study

- This was a single-center, cross-sectional, descriptive study.

II. Study period

Our study took place from January 1, 2021 to December 31, 2022.

III. Study location

-The study took place in the pneumo-paediatrics B department of the Abderrahmen Mami hospital in Ariana.

IV. Study population

1. Inclusion criteria

-Patients under 18 years of age.

-Managed for bronchiolitis obliterans between January 2013 and January 2022.

-With a positive diagnosis of BO based on the following criteria (7) :

-History of severe respiratory infection or bone marrow transplant.

-Bronchial obstruction not improved by bronchodilators or systemic corticosteroids and revealed by clinical symptoms and/or respiratory function tests.

-Aspect of mosaic perfusion or entrapment on thoracic CT.

-Exclusion of other chronic respiratory pathologies: asthma, cystic fibrosis, primary ciliary dyskinesia, bronchopulmonary dysplasia, alpha-1 antitrypsin deficiency and immune deficiency.

2. Non-inclusion criteria

-Patients over 18 years of age.

-Children not diagnosed with BO.

-Children whose parents refused to participate in the study.

3. Exclusion criteria

Children lost to follow-up during the study period.

-Children with associated diffuse infiltrative lung disease.

V. Course of the study

1. Data collection

The following clinical and paraclinical data were taken from the children's medical records:

Date of birth, family respiratory history, personal medical and surgical history, age of onset of symptoms, date of diagnosis of bronchiolitis obliterans, date of start of follow-up in our department, initial functional signs, initial physical examination, data from initial chest CT scan, data from respiratory function tests (if performed), prescribed treatments (molecule, dosage, route of administration, possible side effects, duration), number of hospitalizations for respiratory symptoms, results of bacteriological sampling (if performed), prescription of home oxygen therapy (if performed), data from cardiac ultrasound (if performed).

2. Disease assessment

The children's parents were contacted by telephone and summoned for a clinical and functional check-up according to their availability and after their consent.

-Parents and/or children were asked about functional signs present at the time of this visit, the number of respiratory exacerbations since the last consultation, whether they had used oral corticosteroids and/or antibiotics for respiratory discomfort, compliance with their background BO treatments, and compliance with home oxygen therapy for children with chronic respiratory insufficiency.

-**Dyspnea** was assessed using the Medical Research Council (mMRC) modified dyspnea scale:

0: No dyspnea, except in the event of heavy physical effort.

1 Dyspnea when walking fast on flat ground or slight inclines.

2 Dyspnea when walking on level ground following someone your own age, or having to stop to catch your breath when walking on level ground at your own pace.

3 Dyspnea, requiring you to stop and catch your breath after a few minutes or a hundred meters on flat ground.

4 Dyspnea when dressing or undressing

-Peak expiratory flow (PEF) was measured during this consultation, a simple test in which the child is asked to blow as fast and hard as possible into the PEF meter.

-Then, **spirometry with a bronchodilation test** was performed on the ward according to 2019 ATS/ERS recommendations (8).

Obstructive ventilatory disorder was defined by a FEV1/FVC ratio < lower limit of normal or a Zscore < -1.64. A positive response to bronchodilators was defined by an improvement in FEV1 of more than 10% of the predicted value (9).

A 6-minute walk test was also carried out on the ward by the physiotherapist.

-A favorable evolution was defined by :

The absence of an acute exacerbation of respiratory disease, defined as an increase in respiratory symptoms requiring therapeutic modification or hospitalization, and the absence of a fall in FEV1 according to the Zscore.

VI. Statistical study

Data were entered and analyzed using SPSS version 11.5 software.

We calculated simple frequencies and relative frequencies (percentages) for the categorical variables.

We calculated means and standard deviations and determined extreme values for quantitative variables.

VII. Ethical considerations

We have respected the anonymity of our patients involved in this work.

We obtained written consent from our patients' parents prior to their inclusion.

Our work presents no conflict of interest.

VIII. Bibliographic research

The search engines used were : PubMed, Sciences direct.

Key words used were: Bronchiolitis obliterans, children, lung function, macrolides, prognosis.

References were entered and organized using ZOTERO software.

RESULTS

I. Clinical and paraclinical study at the time of diagnosis

Eighteen children were treated for bronchiolitis obliterans (BO) in our department during the inclusion period (09years).

1. Population characteristics

Age

The mean age was 9.6 years [3-17 years]. Half of the children were under 10 years of age at the time of the study (Figure 1).

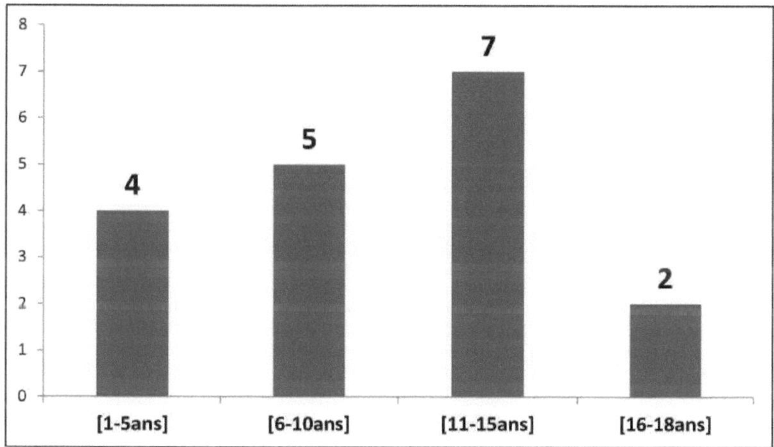

Figure 1: Distribution of children by age

Gender

The sex ratio was 1.5, with 11 boys and 7 girls.

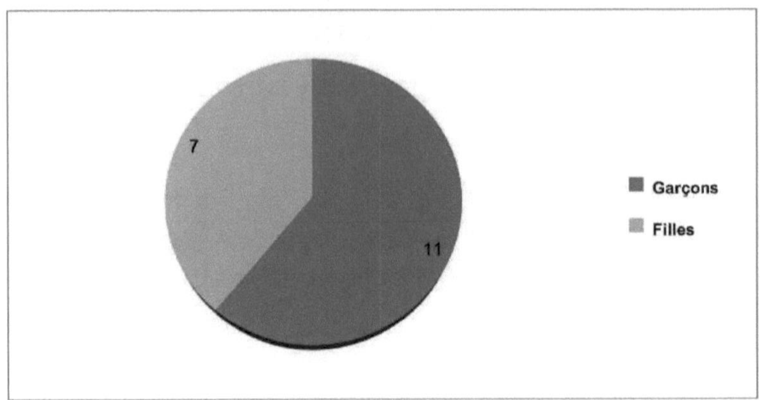

Figure 2: Distribution of children by gender

Pathological history

Twelve children had a history of haemopathy for which a bone marrow transplant was performed (67%) (Table I).

Table I: Indications for bone marrow transplantation in our population

Hemopathy	Workforce
Variable common immune deficiency	3
Acute lymphoblastic leukemia	3
Myelodysplastic syndrome	2
Acute myeloid leukemia	2
Fanconi's disease	1
Sickle cell disease	1

A history of severe respiratory infection prior to BO was present in 6 children (33%). Three children required mechanical ventilation during this infectious episode.

2. Positive diagnosis of bronchiolitis obliterans

Age of positive diagnosis

The mean age at diagnosis of bronchiolitis obliterans was 66 months [12-204 months].

The mean duration of disease progression at the time of the study was 39 months [18-162].

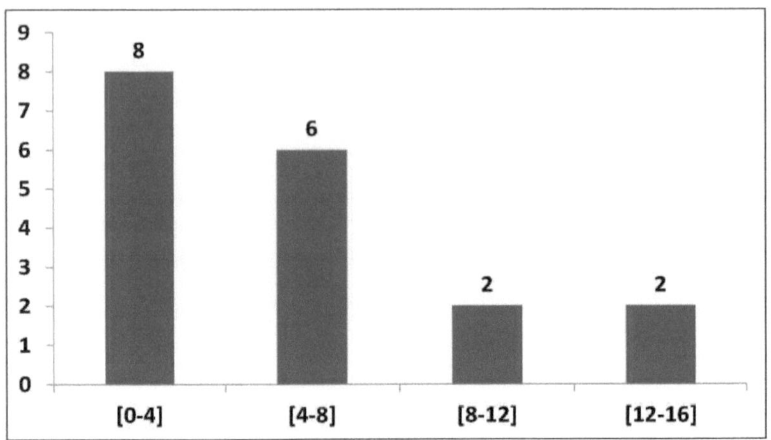

Figure 3: Distribution of children by age of diagnosis

Clinical signs

Dyspnea was present in 100% of children (figure 4). It was wheezing in 12 patients.

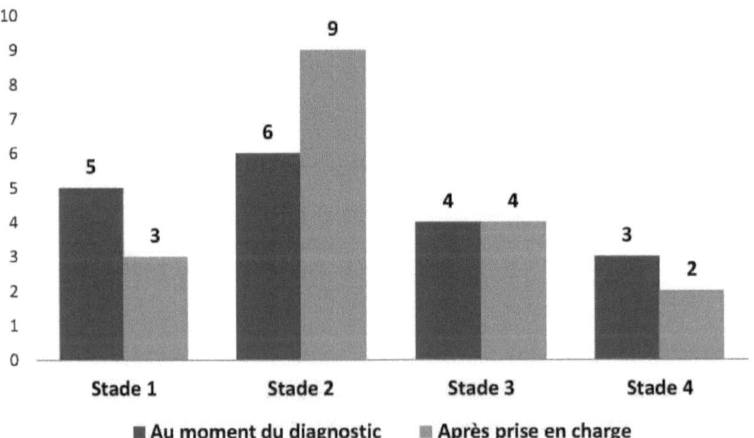

Figure 4: Classification of exertional dyspnea according to mMRC stage

Other functional signs were dominated by cough (94%), recurrent lower respiratory infections (72%), bronchorrhea (22%) and chest pain (16%) (Figure 5).

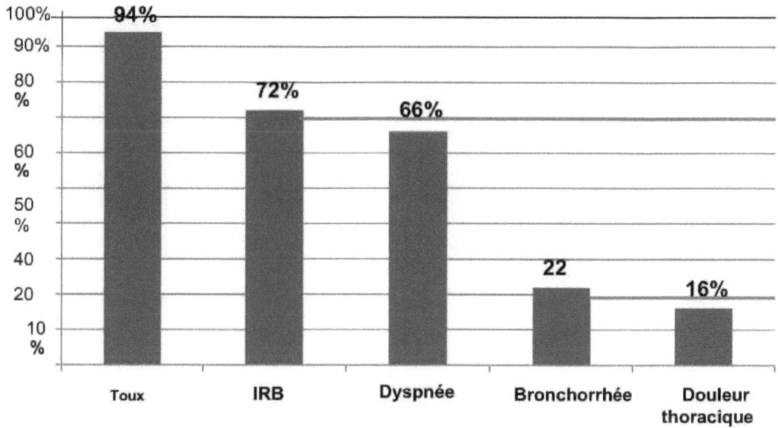

Figure 5: Pulmonary function signs

Mean peripheral oxygen saturation was 93% [88%-98%]. Seven children were initially admitted for acute respiratory failure (38%). Polypnoea was the most frequent physical sign (83%).

Ten children had growth retardation associated with respiratory symptoms (55%). Digital hippocratism and thoracic deformity were observed in 4 children (22%) and 8 children (44%) respectively.

Nine children had sibilant rales on pulmonary auscultation. Peak expiratory flow was measured in 12 children. Its median value was 63% of the theoretical value [21%-88%].

Eight children were in chronic respiratory failure at the time of diagnosis, each requiring 1 liter per minute of long-term oxygen therapy (LTO) (44%).

Thoracic imaging

Chest CT scans were performed in all children at the time of initial diagnosis. Mosaic perfusion was present in all our patients. Figure 6 shows two parenchymal sections of a chest CT scan of a 07-year-old child with post-bone marrow transplant BO.

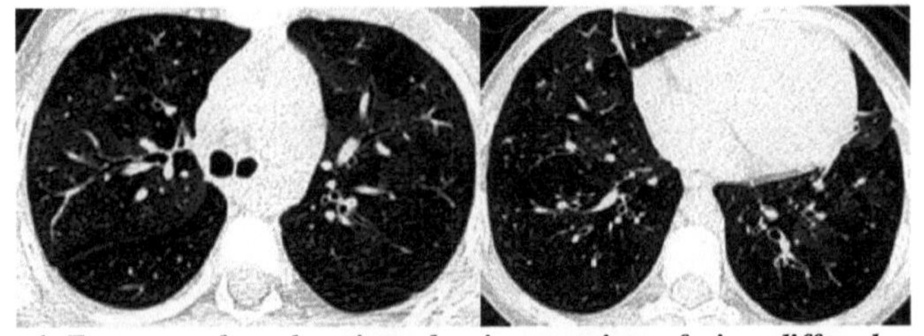

Figure 6: Two parenchymal sections showing mosaic perfusion, diffuse bronchial thickening and mucoid impactions.

Scannographic abnormalities are detailed in Table II.

Table II: Thoracic imaging abnormalities

	Number	*Percentage*
Mosaic infusion	***18***	***100%***
Trapping	***17***	***94%***
Bronchial thickening	***14***	***77%***
DDB	***12***	***67%***
Chest distension	***10***	***55%***
Mucoid impactions	***5***	***27%***
Atelectasis	***4***	***22%***
Dilatation of the pulmonary arteries	***4***	***22%***

Initial respiratory function tests

Spirometry and a bronchodilation test were performed in 13 children prior to initiation of treatment, showing a non-reversible obstructive ventilatory deficit in all cases (Table 3). FEV1 was < -3DS in 12 of the 13 children who were able to perform spirometry.

A fall in FVC from the lower limit of normal was observed in 10 cases.

Plethysmography could not be performed in our population due to a technical problem with the plethysmograph during the study period.

Table III: Spirometry abnormalities

	Before B2 mimetics		After B2 mimetics	
	Percentage	*Z score*	*Percentage*	*Z score*
Median FEV1	*48%*	*-4 [-7.9,-1.6]*	*46%*	*-4.1*
Median FVC	*59%*	*-3 [-4,-1.8]*	*58%*	*-2.8*
FEV1/FVC	*81%*	*-2.5 [-8,-1.64]*	*80%*	*-1.6*

The 6-minute walk test was possible in 6 cases. Arterial desaturation was observed in 50% of cases. The average distance covered was 435m.

3. Etiological diagnosis

Graft-versus-host disease was the most frequent etiology of BO (12 cases). OL was post-infectious in 6 cases (33%) (Figure 7).

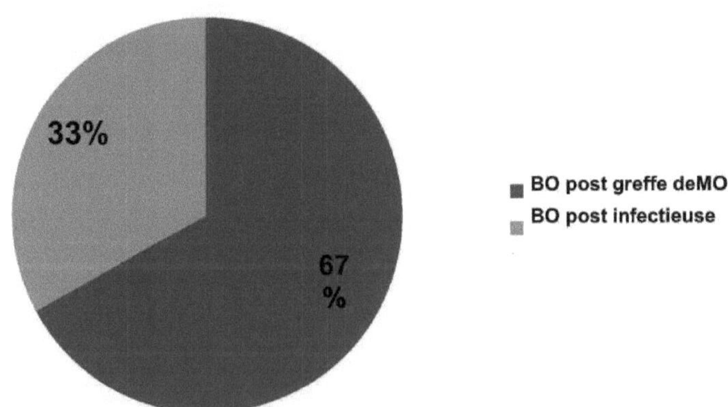

Figure 7: Etiological diagnosis of bronchiolitis obliterans

BO post bone marrow transplant

Mean age of children with BO secondary to graft-versus-host disease (GVH) was 09y ±3.7 [2-17y], with nine boys and three girls.

The average time between bone marrow transplantation and the diagnosis of BO was 15 months [6
36 months]. The mean age at diagnosis of GVH was 7y ±2.9 [1-12y].

A 12-year-old girl required a 2nd bone marrow transplant following a relapse of acute B lymphocytic leukemia. BO was diagnosed 20 months after the second transplant.
Other graft-versus-host disease (GVHD) localizations were cutaneous (5 cases), hepatic (4 cases) and digestive (1 case).

Post-infectious BO:

Six children had post-infectious BO with a mean age of 8÷4 years. The mean age at the time of pulmonary infection was 2y [1-4y]. BO was secondary to adenovirus infection in one boy and one girl. For the rest of the children, the initial bacteriological investigation was negative. Two children had required intubation for the initial respiratory infection.
fl there was no free interval between severe respiratory infection and the onset of bronchiolitis obliterans.

II Child follow-up and clinical and functional development

1 Monitoring children in service

Eight children were referred to us for management of confirmed BO in the setting of pulmonary GVH associated with cutaneous and hepatic GVH.
The diagnosis was suspected in 4 other transplanted children and confirmed in our department.
Non-transplanted children were initially referred to us for respiratory symptoms, and the diagnosis of post-infectious BO was made after clinical, radiological and functional workup.
The mean duration of follow-up in our department was 51 months [16-144 months].

2. Treatments initiated

Inhaled corticosteroids (ICS)

All children were on inhaled corticosteroids with a mean dose of 815ug beclomethasone per day [500-1000]. The mean duration of inhaled corticosteroid therapy was 44 months.

Long-acting bronchodilators (LABA)

Fourteen children were taking LABA in fixed combination with inhaled corticosteroids (78%). The molecule prescribed was salmeterol, and the daily dose was 25ug twice a day.

Anti-leukotrienes

Six children were treated with anti-leukotrienes (33%). Montelukast was available in Tunisia but not in the hospital nomenclature.

Macrolides

Thirteen children were on macrolides (72%). The drug prescribed was azithromycin, taken 1 day in 2 at half dose (dose weight/2 per dose).

Oral corticosteroid therapy

Twelve children were on long-term oral corticosteroid therapy at a mean dose of 0.95mg/kg/day prednisone equivalent [0.5-1.5mg/kg/d] prescribed for GVH. Two other children with post-infectious bronchiolitis obliterans had received monthly courses of methylprednisolone boli for 6 months.

The mean duration of systemic corticosteroid therapy was 46 months [8-67].

During follow-up, 3 children were weaned off oral corticosteroids.

3. Evolution

Clinical course

The clinical course was favorable in 3 patients, with no need for hospitalization, systemic corticosteroids or other complications.

Figure 8 shows the evolution of dyspnoea according to the m MRC stage after treatment.

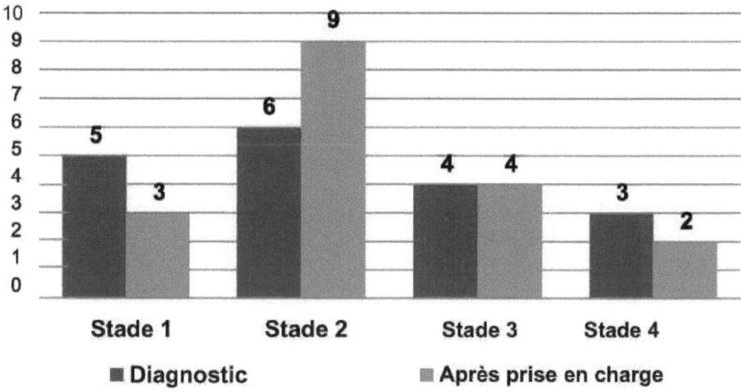

Figure 8: Evolution of exertional dyspnea according to mMRC stage

The evolution of other respiratory symptoms was marked by regression of coughing, nausea and vomiting.

sifflements et des douleurs thoraciques (figure 9).

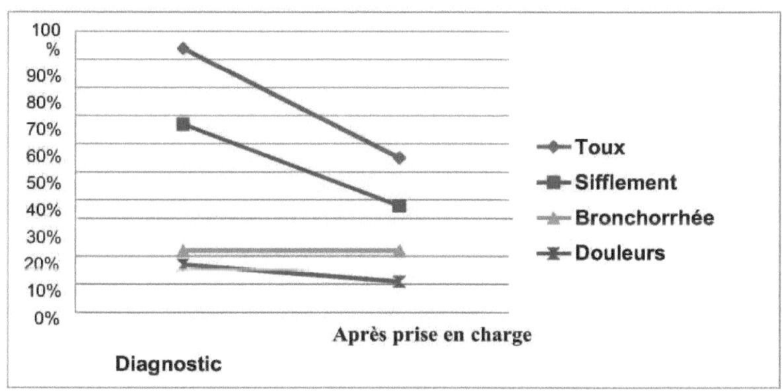

Figure 9: Evolution of respiratory symptoms

Evolution of respiratory function

Seven patients had follow-up spirometry. The absolute value of FEV1 increased during follow-up in 6 children (Figure 8). The mean gain in FEV1 in these children was 85 ml per year.

A decline in FEV1 from 800 ml to 280 ml after 3 years was observed in a 6-year-old boy with BO in the setting of pulmonary, cutaneous and hepatic GVH. This patient required six hospitalizations for acute exacerbations with acute respiratory failure during 03 years of follow-up (Figure 10).

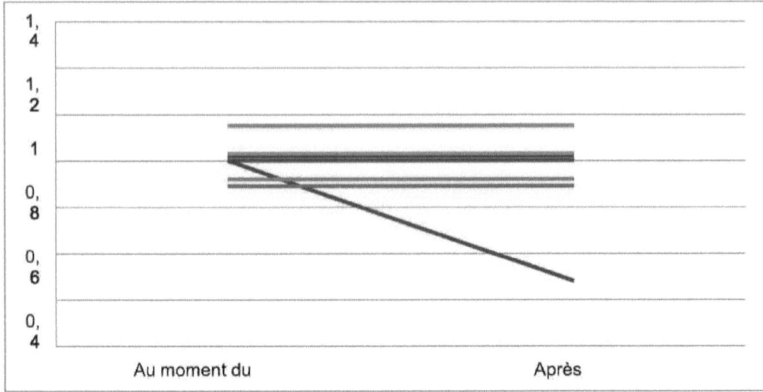

Figure 10: Changes in FEV1 during follow-up (in liters)

According to the Z score, worsening FEV1 was observed in 3 cases (42%). Two patients had stable FEV1 (29%) and 2 patients had improved FEV1 (29%) (Figure 11).

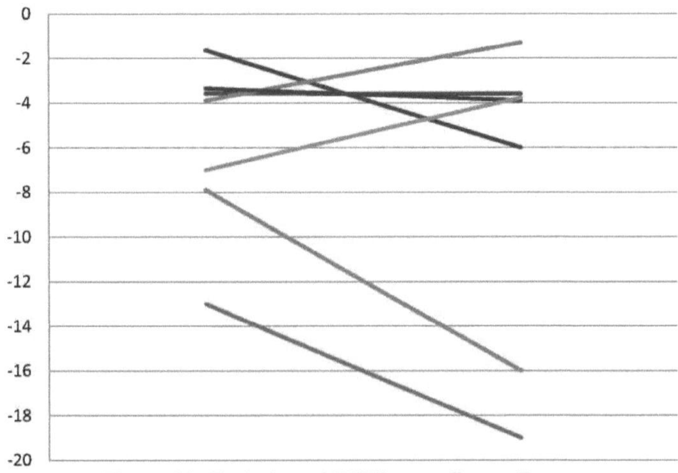

Figure 11: Evolution of FEV1 according to Z-score

4. Complications

Acute exacerbations

The mean number of exacerbations per child was 2.38 [1-7]. The average hospital stay was 2.4 per child [0-7]. Acute respiratory failure was the cause of hospitalization in 90% of cases. Six children required intensive care (33%), with recourse to non-invasive ventilation. Two other children required mechanical ventilation.

The most frequent cause of exacerbation was a lower respiratory infection, observed in 11 children (61%). The germs responsible are shown in figure 12.

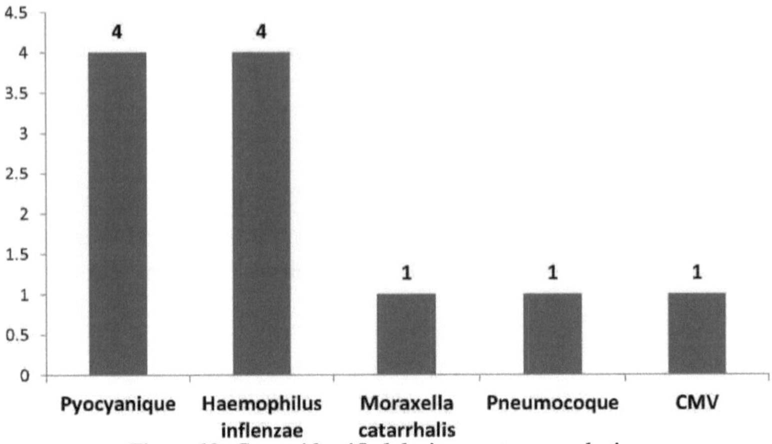

Figure 12: Germs identified during acute exacerbations

Iatrogenicity of prescribed treatments

A child had developed palpitations following initiation of long-acting bronchodilators. The rhythmic holter showed sinus tachycardia which regressed when the B2 mimetics were stopped.

Iatrogenicity was observed in 11 children on long-term oral corticosteroid therapy (figure13).

No side effects were observed with anti-leukotrienes or macrolides in our series. Nevertheless, we opted to discontinue anti-leukotrienes in 2 children who had developed a depressive syndrome.

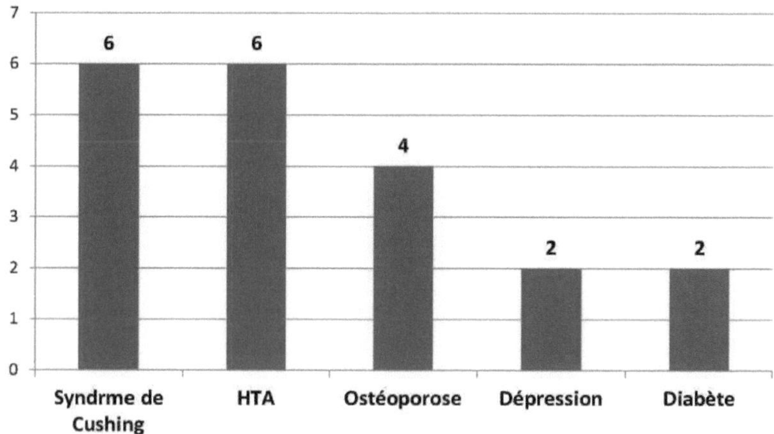

Figure 13: Iatrogenic effects of oral corticosteroids

Chronic respiratory insufficiency

Eight children were on home oxygen therapy at the time of diagnosis (44%). Oxygen weaning was possible in 2 children treated for post-infectious BO.

None of the other children progressed to chronic respiratory failure during the study.

Pulmonary hypertension

Three children had evidence of pulmonary hypertension on cardiac ultrasound, with systemic pulmonary arterial pressures assessed at 40, 42 and 45mmHg respectively.

Pneumothorax

This complication was observed in two children with pulmonary GVH. The 2 children had undergone pleural symphysis, the indications for which were a homolateral recurrence of a left pneumothorax in the first patient and a bilateral pneumothorax in the second patient.

Pleural symphysis was performed through the thoracic drain in the first patient due to a high anesthetic risk associated with chronic respiratory insufficiency. The second patient underwent surgical pleural symphysis under thoracoscopy without incident.

4.7. Deaths

During the course of our study, the follow-up of our patients was marked by the occurrence of death in 2 patients with post-MO transplant BO (11%) with a survival of 27 months for the first patient and 12 months for the second patient.
The cause of death was acute respiratory distress requiring a stay in intensive care and mechanical ventilation in both children.

DISCUSSION

Bronchiolitis obliterans is an anatomopathological entity characterized by inflammatory and fibrosing phenomena of the small airways, with little adjacent lung parenchyma. Diagnostic criteria are essentially clinical, radiological and functional. The most frequent etiologies in children are dominated by graft-versus-host disease and severe respiratory infections, fl there are no clear recommendations for the therapeutic management of this rare entity.

In our study, we collated 18 children diagnosed with bronchiolitis obliterans during the period from January 1[er] 2013 to January 1 2022. Indeed, this is a rare disease often underdiagnosed outside the context of bone marrow transplantation. In a multicenter study conducted in Hong Kong, 56 children were collated over a 19-year period (between 1996 and 2015) (10).

A predominance of the disease in boys has been reported in the literature [11]. The gender ratio in our study was 1.5.

In our series, obliterative bronchiolitis was secondary to bone marrow transplantation in 2/3 of cases, whereas in the study cited above, post-infectious obliterative bronchiolitis (PIOB) was the dominant etiology (10). This may be due to a selection bias, as the national bone marrow transplant center in Tunis refers transplanted children to our consultation with any respiratory symptomatology. Post-infectious BO is most often managed in pediatric wards juxtaposed to pediatric intensive care units. BOPI was secondary to severe adenovirus infection in 2 cases. In the literature, this is one of the most frequently incriminated germs in this pathology, along with respiratory syncitial virus, measles virus and mycoplasma (11). Other risk factors for BOPI reported in previous studies were mechanical ventilation and severe hypoxemia during the infectious episode (12,13).

Bone marrow transplantation has improved the prognosis of several hematological malignancies and benign diseases worldwide and in Tunisia. In our study, the main indications were: acute leukemia, variable common immunodeficiency, myelodysplastic syndrome, Fanconi's disease and sickle cell anemia. Unfortunately, this innovative therapy is a source of significant acute and late complications. In a Tunisian study published in 2017 by the team at the Tunis Bone Marrow Transplant Center, which included 32 patients, the most frequent late complication was graft-versus-host disease (GVHD) observed in 41% of cases, with a care-related cost three times higher (14). Graft versus host disease is the most frequent and formidable pulmonary GVHD (15).

The risk factors reported in the literature for the occurrence of OL post-transplant were: the presence of other GVHD localizations, gender mismatch between donor and recipient, and busulfan conditioning (3,16,17). In our study, ten of the transplanted children had at least one extrapulmonary localization of graft-versus-host disease. The mean time to onset of OL after bone marrow transplantation varies between 12 and 24 months [18]. In our study, the average delay was 15 months [6-36 months].

The mean age at the time of positive diagnosis in our population was 07 years for BO secondary to OM transplantation and 02 years for acute post-infectious bronchiolitis. Our data are consistent with those reported in the literature. Indeed, post-infectious BO is more frequent in young children, given the increased risk of severe respiratory infections during the first three years of life [19].

Dyspnea and cough were the predominant functional signs in our population. Dyspnoea was classified as greater than two according to mMRC in 38% of children. In the study conducted by the Hong Kong team, the same symptoms were observed (10).
Polypnoea was the most frequent sign on physical examination (83%). This sign was almost constant in several other studies (2,10,20). Chest deformity and digital hippocratism were observed in 50% and 22% of cases respectively. In the series by Lino et al, 20% of children had digital hippocratism and 63% thoracic deformity (20). Growth retardation was observed in half of our population (55%). This would be related to the energy expenditure due to excessive respiratory work during the course of this pathology. In the literature, chronic respiratory failure is a frequent complication of BO. In the study by Aguerre et al, which included 52 children with BOPI, 62% were on long-term oxygen therapy at the time of diagnosis (21). In the present study, eight children had chronic respiratory failure requiring home oxygen therapy (44%). Of these, five had pulmonary

GVH and three had post-infectious BO.

Chest CT is a key element in the positive diagnosis of bronchiolitis obliterans. In typical cases, it shows a mosaic perfusion pattern. Jensen et al compared the CT data of patients with BOPI and severe asthmatics. The discriminating abnormality between the 2 groups was mosaic perfusion with $p < 0.006$ (22). Other abnormalities described in previous studies include bronchial thickening, expiratory trapping, atelectasis and bronchiectasis (1,11). All these radiological aspects were observed in our study, with mosaic perfusion present in 100% of cases.

In addition to its contribution to positive diagnosis, some authors have used chest CT to assess the severity of the disease and the degree of bronchial obstruction (23-25). In a Korean study of 17 children with BOPI, the presence of bronchial thickening on CT was associated with a better response to systemic corticosteroid therapy (26). This radiological sign was present in 70% of cases in our series.

Respiratory function tests show non-reversible bronchial obstruction after broncho-dilation testing. Nevertheless, in advanced forms of the disease, a decrease in forced vital capacity (FVC) and a drop in carbon monoxide diffusion capacity can be observed (27-29). Of the 13 children in whom spirometry could be performed at the time of diagnosis, 12 had an obstructive ventilatory disorder with FEV1 <-3SD. Our data concur with those reported in the literature (Table 4). In the majority of cases, the drop in FVC was due to air trapping. Plethysmography often confirms thoracic distension by showing an increase in total lung capacity. However, due to technical problems, this test could not be performed on our patients.

Table IV: Initial FEV1 evaluated by Z-score in the literature

	Number of patients	***Year***	***FEV1 in Z-score***
Jung J (30)	***47***	***2021***	***-2 [-2.4 , -1.6]***
Kim J (23)	***23***	***2019***	***-2.2 [-3.5 , -1.2]***
Mattiello R (31)	***72***	***2016***	***-4 [-4.4 ,-3.6]***
Colom A (28)	***46***	***2015***	***-4.3 [-4.6 ,-4.0]***
Our study	***18***	***2023***	***-4.1 [-7.9,-1.6]***

Respiratory function monitoring is based on the measurement of forced expiratory volume in one second (FEV1). Early and rapid decline in FEV1 is associated with a poorer prognosis (32). In our population, 42% of children showed a decline in FEV1 according to the Z-score during follow-up. Two of these children died.
In a Korean study of 82 children with post-bone marrow transplant BO, FEV1 below 30% of predicted value was predictive of mortality, with a mean survival of 23.7 months versus 48.4 months in children with FEV1 above 30% (33).

Histological signature is not part of the diagnostic criteria for bronchiolitis obliterans, whether post-transplant or following severe respiratory infection (34). Indeed, given the vulnerability of these patients and their limited respiratory function, lung biopsy is often avoided. It may be indicated in cases of atypical clinical presentation with associated diffuse infiltrative lung disease, if other non-invasive investigations prove inconclusive. In our study, a single lung biopsy was performed under thoracoscopy in a patient presenting with bilateral pneumothorax. The main indication for surgery was pleural symphysis.

In addition to pneumothorax, bronchiolitis obliterans can lead to other complications, such as respiratory exacerbations. These are most often of infectious origin (35). Recurrent pulmonary infections are associated with a poorer prognosis (36). In our study, 61% of acute exacerbations were of infectious origin. The causative germs identified were: pseudomonas Aerauginosa and EHaemophilus Influenzae, followed by pneumococcus and Moraxella Catarrhalis. Our data concur with those reported in the literature (36). Indeed, in a Japanese study published in 2020, pyocyanins were the most frequent germ in bacteriological samples taken from patients with BO (36).

There are no current recommendations for the therapeutic management of bronchiolitis obliterans. In fact, several therapies have been tried by different teams in retrospective or prospective studies. Most of these studies involved small numbers of children, making it impossible to establish a universal therapeutic consensus. The most commonly used drugs were corticosteroids, long-acting bronchodilators, macrolides and anti-leukotrienes (1,5).

Systemic corticosteroid therapy is one of the most widely prescribed treatments for both graft-versus-host disease and post-infectious bronchiolitis obliterans, especially in the early phase of the disease.
Studies of histopathological patterns have shown that the degree of inflammation and peribronchiolar fibrosis is subject to inter-individual variation (37). According to some authors, the lymphocytic cell profile may be a predictive factor for a favorable response to lacorticotherapy (38).
There is no consensus on the route of administration or dosage of corticosteroids. Some authors prefer the inhaled route, which minimizes the occurrence of adverse effects. Others suggest that aerosol deposition of inhaled corticosteroids is minimal in the affected bronchioles, which may compromise their efficacy (39).
A therapeutic protocol including monthly boli of high-dose intravenous methylprednisolone reduced the frequency of exacerbations and improved respiratory function (40-43). Nevertheless, this corticosteroid therapy has been associated with several iatrogenic complications such as osteoporosis, arterial hypertension, increased infectious risk and hyperglycemia (40). In the present study, Ilenfants had developed complications secondary to the prescription of corticosteroids.

In the study by Zhang et al published in 2018, 30 children with post-infectious bronchiolitis obliterans were put on combination nebulizations of budesonide, terbutaline and ipratropium bromide for one year. Subsequent follow-up showed significant improvement in symptom score, lung function and mosaic perfusion CT images (44).

Treatment with inhaled bronchodilators appears to improve functional signs and quality of life in some BO patients who retain a positive response after bronchodilation testing. A Brazilian study published in 2016 that included 72 children followed up for BOPI showed a positive bronchodilation test in 47.2% with reference to the 2005 ATS/ERS recommendations, i.e. a 12% increase in FEV1 after inhalation of B2 mimetics (31).

Long-term use of macrolides has become increasingly widespread in a number of chronic respiratory diseases since the discovery of their anti-inflammatory effect (45). A reduction in neutrophil and eosinophil activity, as well as a decrease in certain inflammatory cytokines, have been demonstrated following macrolide treatment (46,47). In a randomized controlled trial (25 azithromycin, 23 placebo), published in 2015 and enrolling post-lung transplant BO patients, a significant gain in FEV1 was observed (48). In our study, we did not note any side effects associated with the prescription of macrolides. However, several complications have been described in the literature, the most frequent of which are the risk of mycobacterial infection, cardiac toxicity and liver toxicity (49-51). Monitoring of these side effects is recommended for patients on long-term macrolide therapy.

Following the premature termination of the randomized double-blind clinical trial (azithromycin versus placebo) due to the increased risk of death from hematological relapse in the azithromycin group, the use of macrolides in children who have undergone bone marrow transplantation for hematological malignancies has been curtailed (52).

Isolated cases of ninedanib efficacy have been reported in the setting of bronchiolitis obliterans associated with diffuse infiltrative lung disease (53). We excluded patients presenting with this entity in the present study, given its clinical, functional and radiological particularities, which may present a selection bias.

In a Chinese study published in 2021 and involving 54 children followed up for BOPI, a protocol combining budesonide, azithromycin, montelukast and acetylcysteine was administered to 54 children for 3 months. Progression was marked by a significant reduction in respiratory symptoms (cough, wheezing, dyspnoea). Chest imaging showed regression of bronchial thickening, atelectasis and mosaic perfusion. No treatment-related adverse events were reported in the same study (54).

In a multicenter study of 36 patients with post-bone marrow transplant BO, a combination of fluticasone, azithromycin and montelukast was prescribed for 06 months. The authors

concluded that this protocol slowed the decline in respiratory function and subsequently improved patients' quality of life (5).
Our department's approach to the management of BO follows this protocol, with a combination of inhaled corticosteroids, anti-leukotrienes and macrolides in the absence of any contraindications. Long-acting bronchodilators are prescribed from the age of four.

In our context, only inhaled corticosteroids and LABAs are available in the hospital nomenclature. As a result, compliance with anti-leukotriene and macrolide therapy was not achieved.
On the other hand, macrolides could not be prescribed for children with a history of haematological malignancy, given the risk of neoplastic relapse.
Also, the psychological problems associated with the chronic course of the disease and recurrent hospitalizations prompted 2 patients to stop taking anti-leukotrienes.

Follow-up of our patients showed a mortality rate of 11%. This rate is close to that described in the literature. The two children who died in our series had graft-versus-host disease. The prognosis of this post-bone marrow transplant complication remains poor, even in developed countries (4). In addition to the natural progression of bronchiolitis obliterans to chronic respiratory failure and pulmonary hypertension, morbidity and mortality are also due to the adverse effects of systemic corticosteroid therapy and the various immunosuppressive treatments prescribed over the long term. The weakening of patients' immune defenses by these therapies makes them vulnerable to all types of infection.

Clinical improvement with weaning from long-term oxygen therapy was possible in 2 children with post-infectious bronchiolitis obliterans. The prognosis of this entity varies from study to study (26,30,39). Some studies suggest that clinical improvement is possible because lung development and alveolization continue throughout childhood and even adolescence (55).

Our study has certain limitations due to its monocentric nature, with a small patient

sample that does not allow comparison of patient subgroups.
Despite its limitations, our study has enabled us to investigate a serious pathology which mainly affects children and young subjects, and which is becoming an increasing concern in our country. On the one hand, bone marrow transplantation has become standard practice, enabling the treatment of hematological malignancies in children, as well as some congenital hemopathies (sickle cell anemia and certain immune deficiencies). On the other hand, advances in ventilation techniques in paediatric intensive care units have improved the survival of severe respiratory infections in children, but long-term sequelae are still observed.

At the end of this study, we propose the following measures:

Establish a respiratory follow-up protocol for children undergoing bone marrow transplantation: a clinical examination, thoracic imaging and respiratory function tests pre-transplant, followed by respiratory and functional follow-up every three months after bone marrow transplantation. This will enable early detection of post-bone marrow transplant BO.

Urge primary care physicians and specialists to follow up children after respiratory infections until all clinical and radiological abnormalities have disappeared, in order to detect post-infectious BO.

-When faced with a diagnosis of bronchiolitis obliterans, a protocol combining inhaled corticosteroid therapy, an anti-leukotriene and a macrolide may be tried, provided there are no contraindications and the benefit-risk balance is continuously monitored.

-Cures of systemic corticosteroid therapy may be proposed during exacerbations, after taking into account the risk of infection.

-Infectious exacerbations should be treated with antibiotic therapy, which will be adapted at a later date depending on the results of bacteriological sampling.

CONCLUSIONS

Bronchiolitis obliterans is a serious chronic respiratory disease with a high morbidity and mortality rate. Diagnosis is based on clinical, radiological and functional criteria. In typical cases, CT scans show mosaic perfusion, expiratory trapping and bronchial thickening. Spirometry shows fixed bronchial obstruction. Histological signature is rarely indicated, given the difficulty of obtaining lung samples from these often vulnerable patients. Its etiologies in children are dominated by sequelae of severe respiratory infection and graft-versus-host disease (GVHD). When it is of post-infectious origin, this entity is still under-diagnosed due to the difficulties of performing functional explorations in this age group. In the context of bone marrow transplantation, however, diagnosis is often straightforward, especially when associated with other GVH localizations. The absence of a universal therapeutic consensus makes its management more difficult. Several protocols have been reported in the literature, with controversial results

On the one hand, the small number of children included in previous studies makes it impossible to establish recommendations. On the other hand, the disease has been shown to be characterized by phenotypic polymorphism. Studies of the disease's clusters and endotypes are currently underway, with a view to developing personalized treatments for each patient.

The aim of our study was to investigate the clinical and paraclinical profile of children followed in our department for obliterative bronchiolitis and to assess the impact of our management on the clinical and functional prognosis of the disease.

This real-life study highlighted the high morbidity and mortality associated with this pathology in our context, and illustrated the difficulties of diagnostic and therapeutic management.

Prevention of severe respiratory infections through barrier measures and vaccination reduces the incidence of long-term sequelae. Systematic respiratory monitoring of children after bone marrow transplants enables early detection of late pulmonary complications.

REFERENCES

1. Kavaliunaite E, Aurora P. Diagnosing and managing bronchiolitis obliterans in children. Expert Review of Respiratory Medicine. May 4, 2019;13(5):481-8.

2. Moonnumakal SP, Fan LL. Bronchiolitis obliterans in children. Current Opinion in Pediatrics. June 2008;20(3):272-8.

3. Bergeron A, Godet C, Chevret S, Lorillon G, Peffault de Latour R, de Revel T, et al. Bronchiolitis obliterans syndrome after allogeneic hematopoietic SCT: phenotypes and prognosis. Bone Marrow Transplant. 2013;48(6):819-24.

4. Hakim A, Cooke KR, Pavletic SZ, Khalid M, Williams KM, Hashmi SK. Diagnosis and treatment of bronchiolitis obliterans syndrome universally accessible. Bone Marrow Transplant. March 2019;54(3):383-92.

5. Williams KM, Cheng GS, Pusic I, Jagasia M, Burns L, Ho VT, et al. FAM treatment for new onset bronchiolitis obliterans syndrome after hematopoietic cell transplantation. Biol Blood Marrow Transplant. Apr 2016;22(4):710-6.

6. Direct cost analysis of the second year post-allogeneic hematopoietic stem cell transplantation in the Bone Marrow Transplant Centre of Tunisia [Internet]. [cited 28 Jan 2023]. Available from: https://www.tandfonline.com/doi/epdf/10.1080/20016689.2017.1335161?needAccess=tru e&role=button

7. Meyer KC, Raghu G, Verleden GM, Corris PA, Aurora P, Wilson KC, et al. An international ISHLT/ATS/ERS clinical practice guideline: diagnosis and management of bronchiolitis obliterans syndrome. Eur Respir J. Dec 2014;44(6):1479-503.

8. Standardization of Spirometry 2019 Update. An Official American Thoracic Society and European Respiratory Society Technical Statement [Internet]. [cited 29 Jan 2023]. Available from: https://www.atsjournals.org/doi/epdf/10.1164/rccm.201908-1590ST?role=tab

9. Stanojevic S, Kaminsky DA, Miller MR, Thompson B, Aliverti A, Barjaktarevic I, et al. ERS/ATS technical standard on interpretive strategies for routine lung function tests. Eur Respir J. Jul 2022;60(1):2101499.

10. Chan KC, Yu MW, Cheung TWY, Lam DSY, Leung TNH, Tsui TK, et al. Childhood bronchiolitis obliterans in Hong Kong-case series over a 20-year period. Pediatric Pulmonology. 2021;56(l):153-61.

11. Colom AJ, Teper AM. Post-infectious bronchiolitis obliterans. Pediatr Pulmonol. Dec 12, 2018;ppul.24221.

12. Colom AJ, Teper AM, Vollmer WM, Diette GB. Risk factors for the development of bronchiolitis obliterans in children with bronchiolitis. Thorax. June 2006;61(6):503-6.

13. Wu PQ, Li X, Jiang WH, Yin GQ, Lei AH, Xiao Q, et al. Hypoxemia is an independent predictor of bronchiolitis obliterans following respiratory adenoviral infection in children. Springerplus. 20 Sep 2016;5(1):1622.

14. Razgallah Khrouf M, Achour L, Thabti A, Soussi MA, Abdejelil N, Lazreg O, et al. Direct cost analysis of the second year post-allogeneic hematopoietic stem cell transplantation in the Bone Marrow Transplant Centre of Tunisia. J Mark Access Health Policy. 15 June 2017;5(1):1335161.

15. Bergeron A. Late-Onset Noninfectious Pulmonary Complications After Allogeneic Hematopoietic Stem Cell Transplantation. Clinics in Chest Medicine. June 2017;38(2):249-62.

16. Williams KM. Bronchiolitis Obliterans After Allogeneic Hematopoietic Stem Cell Transplantation. JAMA. 15 Jul 2009;302(3):306.

17. Gazourian L, Rogers AJ, Ibanga R, Weinhouse GL, Pinto-Plata V, Ritz J, et al. Factors associated with bronchiolitis obliterans syndrome and chronic graft-versus-host disease after allogeneic hematopoietic cell transplantation. Am J Hematol. Apr 2014;89(4):404-9.

18. Michelson PH, Goyal R, Kurland G. Pulmonary complications of haematopoietic cell transplantation in children. Paediatric Respiratory Reviews. March 1, 2007;8(l):46-61.

19. Liu D, Liu J, Zhang L, Chen Y, Zhang Q. Risk Factors for Post-infectious Bronchiolitis Obliterans in Children: A Systematic Review and Meta-Analysis. Front Pediatr. June 9, 2022;10:881908.

20. Lino CA, Batista AKM, Soares MAD, Filho JHM, Gomes VCC. Bronchiolitis obliterans: clinical and radiological profile of children followed-up in a reference outpatient clinic.

21. Aguerre V, Castaños C, Pena HG, Grenoville M, Murtagh P. Postinfectious bronchiolitis obliterans in children: Clinical and pulmonary function findings. Pediatr Pulmonol. Dec 2010;45(12):118O-5.

22. Jensen SP, Lynch DA, Brown KK, Wenzel SE, Newell JD. High-resolution CT Features of Severe Asthma and Bronchiolitis Obliterans. Clinical Radiology. Dec 2002;57(12):1078-85.

23. Kim J, Kim MJ, Sol IS, Sohn MH, Yoon H, Shin HJ, et al. Quantitative CT and pulmonary function in children with post-infectious bronchiolitis obliterans. PLoS One. Apr 1, 2019;14(4):e0214647.

24. Mattiello R, Sarria EE, Mallol J, Fischer GB, Mocelin H, Bello R, et al. Post-infectious bronchiolitis obliterans: Can CT scan findings at early age anticipate lung function?: CT Findings and Lung Function in PIBO. Pediatr Pulmonol. avr2010;45(4):315-9.

25. Moutafidis D, Gavra M, Golfinopoulos S, Oikonomopoulou C, Kitra V, Woods JC, et al. Lung hyperinflation quantitated by chest CT in children with bronchiolitis obliterans syndrome following allogeneic hematopoietic cell transplantation. Clinical Imaging. Jul 2021;75:97-104.

26. Yoon HM, Lee JS, Hwang JY, Cho YA, Yoon HK, Yu J, et al. Post-infectious bronchiolitis obliterans in children: CT features that predict responsiveness to pulse methylprednisolone. Br J Radiol. May 2015;88(1049):20140478.

27. Barker AF, Bergeron A, Rom WN, Hertz MI. Obliterative Bronchiolitis. N Engl J Med. May 8, 2014;370(19):1820-8.

28. Colom AJ, Maffey A, Garcia Bournissen F, Teper A. Pulmonary function of a paediatric cohort of patients with postinfectious bronchiolitis obliterans. A long term follow-up. Thorax. feb 2015;70(2):169-74.

29. Lee E, Park S, Yang HJ. Pulmonary Function in Post-Infectious Bronchiolitis Obliterans in Children: A Systematic Review and Meta-Analysis. Pathogens. Dec

2022;11(12):1538.

30. Jung JH, Kim GE, Min IK, Jang H, Kim SY, Kim MJ, et al. Prediction of postinfectious bronchiolitis obliterans prognosis in children. Pediatric Pulmonology. May 2021;56(5):1069-76.

31. Mattiello R, Vidal PC, Sarria EE, Pitrez PM, Stein RT, Mocelin HT, et al. Evaluating bronchodilator response in pediatric patients with post-infectious bronchiolitis obliterans: use of different criteria for identifying airway reversibility. J Bras Pneumol. 2016;42(3):174-8.

32. Walther S, Rettinger E, Maurer HM, Pommerening H, Jarisch A, Sorensen J, et al. Longterm pulmonary function testing in pediatric bronchiolitis obliterans syndrome after hematopoietic stem cell transplantation. Pediatric Pulmonology. 2020;55(7):1725-35.

33. Ahn JH, Jo KW, Song JW, Shim TS, Lee SW, Lee JS, et al. Prognostic role of FEV $_1$ for survival in bronchiolitis obliterans syndrome after allogeneic hematopoietic stem cell transplantation. Clin Transplant. dec 2015;29(12):1133-9.

34. Glanville AR, Benden C, Bergeron A, Cheng GS, Gottlieb J, Lease ED, et al. Bronchiolitis obliterans syndrome after lung or haematopoietic stem cell transplantation: current management and future directions. ERJ Open Res. 25 Jul 2022;8(3):00185-2022.

35. Atag E, Bas Ikizoglu N, Ergenekon P, Kalin S, Unal F, Gokdemir Y, et al. Health-related quality of life in patients with bronchiolitis obliterans. Pediatric Pulmonology. Sept 2020;55(9):2361-7.

36. Yomota M, Yanagawa N, Sakai F, Yamada Y, Sekiya N, Ohashi K, et al. Association between chronic bacterial airway infection and prognosis of bronchiolitis obliterans syndrome after hematopoietic cell transplantation. Medicine (Baltimore). Jan 4, 2019;98(1):e13951.

37. Mauad T, Dolhnikoff M, and the S^ko Paulo Bronchiolitis Obliterans Study Group. Histology of childhood bronchiolitis obliterans. Pediatr Pulmonol. June

2002;33(6):466-74.

38. Mauad T, van Schadewijk A, Schrumpf J, Hack CE, Fernezlian S, Garippo AL, et al. Lymphocytic inflammation in childhood bronchiolitis obliterans. Pediatr Pulmonol. Sept 2004;38(3):233-9.

39. Zhang L, Irion K, Kozakewich H, Reid L, Camargo JJ, Porto N da S, et al. Clinical course of postinfectious bronchiolitis obliterans. Pediatr Pulmonol. May 2000;29(5):341-50.

40. Tomikawa SO, Adde FV, da Silva Filho LVRF, Leone C, Rodrigues JC. Follow-up on pediatric patients with bronchiolitis obliterans treated with corticosteroid pulse therapy. Orphanet J Rare Dis. August 15, 2014;9:128.

41. Tanou K, Xaidara A, Kaditis AG. Efficacy of pulse methylprednisolone in a pediatric case of postinfectious bronchiolitis obliterans: Efficacy of Methylprednisolone in Bronchiolitis.

Obliterans. Pediatr Pulmonol. May 2015;50(5):E13-6.

42. Ratjen F, Rjabko O, Kremens B. High-dose corticosteroid therapy for bronchiolitis obliterans after bone marrow transplantation in children. Bone Marrow Transplant. July 2005;36(2):135-8.

43. Even-Or E, Ghandourah H, Ali M, Krueger J, Sweezey NB, Schechter T. Efficacy of high-dose steroids for bronchiolitis obliterans syndrome post pediatric hematopoietic stem cell transplantation. Pediatr Transplantation. march 2018;22(2):e13155.

44. Zhang XM, Lu AZ, Yang HW, Qian LL, Wang LB, Zhang XB. Clinical features of postinfectious bronchiolitis obliterans in children undergoing long-term nebulization treatment. World J Pediatr. Oct 2018;14(5):498-503.

45. Long-term, low-dose macrolide antibiotic treatment in pediatric chronic airway diseases - PMC [Internet]. [cited 15 Apr 2023]. Available from: https://www.ncbi.nlm.nih.gov/pmc/articles/PMC9122820/

46. Brusselle GG, Joos G. Is there a role for macrolides in severe asthma: Current Opinion in Pulmonary Medicine. jan 2014;20(l):95-102.

47. Verleden GM, Vanaudenaerde BM, Dupont LJ, Van Raemdonck DE. Azithromycin

reduces airway neutrophilia and interleukin-8 in patients with bronchiolitis obliterans syndrome. Am J Respir Crit Care Med. 1 Sep 2006;174(5):566-70.

48. Corris PA, Ryan VA, Small T, Lordan J, Fisher AJ, Meachery G, et al. A randomised controlled trial of azithromycin therapy in bronchiolitis obliterans syndrome (BOS) post lung transplantation. Thorax. May 2015;70(5):442-50.

49. Ray WA, Murray KT, Hall K, Arbogast PG, Stein CM. Azithromycin and the Risk of Cardiovascular Death. N Engl J Med. May 17, 2012;366(20):1881-90.

50. Renna M, Schaffner C, Brown K, Shang S, Tamayo MH, Hegyi K, et al. Azithromycin blocks autophagy and may predispose cystic fibrosis patients to mycobacterial infection. J Clin Invest. Sep 1, 2011;121(9):3554-63.

51. Leitner JM, Graninger W, Thalhammer F. Hepatotoxicity of Antibacterials: Pathomechanisms and Clinical Data. Infection. Feb 1, 2010;38(l):3-ll.

52. Bergeron A, Chevret S, Granata A, Chevallier P, Vincent L, Huynh A, et al. Effect of Azithromycin on Airflow Decline-Free Survival After Allogeneic Hematopoietic Stem Cell Transplant: The ALLOZITHRO Randomized Clinical Trial. JAMA. August 8, 2017;318(6):557.

53. Tang W, Yu T, Dong T, Liu T, Ji J. Nintedanib in Bronchiolitis Obliterans Syndrome After Allogeneic Hematopoietic Stem Cell Transplantation. Chest. Sept 2020;158(3):e89-91.

54. Weng T, Lin X, Wang L, Lv J, Dong L. Follow-up on the therapeutic effects of a budesonide, azithromycin, montelukast, and acetylcysteine (BAMA) regimen in children with post-infectious bronchiolitis obliterans. J Thorac Dis. August 2021;13(8):4775-84.

55. Narayanan M, Owers-Bradley J, Beardsmore CS, Mada M, Ball I, Garipov R, et al. Alveolarization Continues during Childhood and Adolescence. Am J Respir Crit Care Med. 15 Jan 2012;185(2):186-91.

Summary

Introduction :

The aim of our work was to study the clinical and paraclinical profile of children followed for obliterative bronchiolitis and to assess the impact of our management on their clinical and functional prognosis.

Methods :

Descriptive cross-sectional study including 18 children managed for bronchiolitis obliterans between January 2013 and December 2021.

Results :

The mean age was 9.6 years [3-17 years], with a male predominance (gender-ratio=1.5). Bronchiolitis obliterans were post-infectious in 33% of cases and post-bone marrow transplant in 67%. Eight children were in chronic respiratory failure at the time of diagnosis. All patients were on inhaled corticosteroids combined with long-acting bronchodilators in 77% of cases, anti-leukotrienes in 33% and macrolides in 72%. The mean duration of follow-up was 51 months [16144 months]. The mean number of hospitalizations was 2.38 per year. The evolution was marked by weaning from long-term oxygen therapy in two children, stability in seven and worsening in six, with two deaths.

Conclusion:

Bronchiolitis obliterans is responsible for significant morbidity and mortality. Management is characterized by a lack of consensus recommendations. Delayed diagnosis and lack of resources are factors that worsen the prognosis in developing countries.

Keywords: Bronchiolitis, infection, transplant, corticosteroid therapy, child

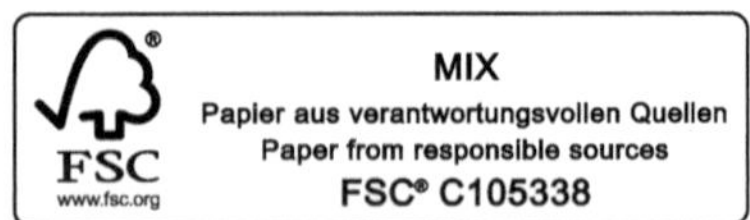

Printed by Books on Demand GmbH, Norderstedt / Germany